HANDBOOK OF
ESSENTIAL INFORMATION
FOR
HOSPITAL DENTAL LEADERS

HANDBOOK OF
ESSENTIAL INFORMATION
FOR
HOSPITAL DENTAL LEADERS

*Arthur I. Hazlewood, DDS, MPH,
FACD, FAAHD, FADI (Hon),
DABSCD*

Chairman Emeritus

*Our Lady of Mercy Medical Center,
Bronx, N.Y.*

iUniverse, Inc.
New York Lincoln Shanghai

HANDBOOK OF ESSENTIAL INFORMATION FOR HOSPITAL DENTAL LEADERS

iUniverse books may be ordered through booksellers or by contacting:

iUniverse
2021 Pine Lake Road, Suite 100
Lincoln, NE 68512
www.iuniverse.com
1-800-Authors (1-800-288-4677)

Because of the dynamic nature of the Internet, any Web addresses or links contained in this book may have changed since publication and may no longer be valid.

The information, ideas, and suggestions in this book are not intended as a substitute for professional medical advice. Before following any suggestions contained in this book, you should consult your personal physician. Neither the author nor the publisher shall be liable or responsible for any loss or damage allegedly arising as a consequence of your use or application of any information or suggestions in this book.

ISBN: 978-0-595-46883-6 (pbk)
ISBN: 978-0-595-91172-1 (ebk)

Printed in the United States of America

Contents

PREFACE

This handbook, which I hope Administrators, Directors, potential Directors and staff will find useful, is based on almost forty years of management experience in the health care sector as Assistant Commissioner of Health, (Bureau Chief), Medical Director and President of the Medical Staff, Dental Director Consultant, the local, state and federal government, as an Executive Board Member, (private non-profit sector.)

This work is based on findings and information derived from observations, discussions, serving as a surveyor and more than thirty years, as a program reviewer and program developer, manager/administrator, teacher and chairman in the hospital arena.

My current role as consultant has provided additional insights. Recently appointed Program Directors and Managers have requested information and guidance in performing their duties. This handbook uses a conceptual and strategic approach. The recommendations are based on established principles, common practice and regulatory requirements so as to apply to the broadest spectrum of institutions. Recommendations based on the author's experience are included. The appendices include some sample documents, but the handbook is not intended to serve as a "cookbook" or operations manual. This edition should be viewed as a primer which provides an overview of leadership responsibilities.

The purpose of the book is to provide the reader with fundamental information required to effectively lead a dental department in a hospital setting. It may also prove useful to anyone interested in the hospital as a location for training and delivery of dental services in the twenty-first century.

The handbook is divided into four sections, plus an appendix, a substantial list of resources and suggested readings.

The first section describes the role of the hospital as an institution. It traces the evolution of the hospital through four major stages dating back to the mid-eighteenth century and bringing it up to the present. Its purpose is to cite the evolution of hospitals from its early beginnings as a refuge to its current stage as a corporate entity. It is intended to provide a context for the discussion and recommendations which follow in the subsequent sections. It briefly describes the changing role of the medical staff over time.

The second section covers the legal structure, organization and governance of hospitals. It includes descriptions of the administration and selected support services.

In the third section entitled Medical/Dental Staff, a wide variety of topics is discussed. The role and characteristics of effective leadership is explored. The Chairman's role, the processes of leadership, strategic planning and credentialing are key topics.

Section four deals exclusively with the operation of the dental department and its relationships with the medical staff, administration, other departments, recruitment, financial management and curriculum development.

ACKNOWLEDGEMENTS

I would like to extend special thanks to Silvestro Iomazzo and Deborah Pasquale for their seminal role in inspiring this handbook. Without their insistence it may never have been written.

My thanks to Dr. Stephen Hancocks (UK) for his patient and helpful advice.

To Lucitta Edwards, I am grateful for her skill, patience, time spent deciphering my scrawl and producing from it a readable manuscript.

My wife Paula is recognized as a willing advisor, listener and a patient reviewer.

Especially I am thankful to Drs. Al Brettner, Carlton Horbelt, Dara Rosenberg, Barry Weinberg and Ms. Carolyn Snipes, who generously gave their thoughtful comments.

Once again my thanks go out to the above-named persons.

SECTION 1
GLOSSARY

COMPETENCY:

Written statement describing levels of knowledge, skills and values expected of a resident completing the program.

DEPARTMENT OF DENTISTRY:

Dental Department = Dental Medicine used interchangeably

GOALS:

Statements of desired outcomes written in very broad but measurable terms

MATCH:

Refers to a system run by a private corporation which establishes a uniform data of appointment to residency programs. It attempts also to match each applicant with his/her highest choice, skills and values expected of trainees completing the program.

MISSION STATEMENT:

Is a statement of purpose of the department. It identifies its target population, services to be provided, addresses issues of quality, and establishes the values on which activities are based. The statement should describe both long-term and short-term actions. It may also include different measures of success such as financial, customer satisfaction, internal operations and staff development.

OBJECTIVES:

More specific performance measures achieved after instruction. They are measurable in both quantitative and behavioral terms.

PASS:

The Postdoctoral Application Support Service (PASS) simplifies the Residency application process. It uses a standardized format which permits applicants to apply to multiple institutions.

PROFICIENCY:

Written statement describing the level of knowledge, skills and values attained when a particular activity is accomplished in more complex situations with repeated quality and a more efficient utilization of time.

VISION STATEMENT:

A picture of the department in the future. It is the starting point for strategic planning and can be a source of motivation

SECTION I

HOSPITAL MISSION AND SERVICE

Section 1

Purpose:

This handbook is based on the premise that the hospital environment is constantly changing and evolving. It is an increasingly complex environment. Financing health care and the management of hospital budgets, continue to be a challenge. Programmatic changes involving new technology are ongoing, as are cost-reducing shifts in programs developed, often in response to changing regulations. As a consequence, the role of department chairpersons in hospitals requires individuals who are knowledgeable, efficient and competent. Department survival may depend on the competence and effectiveness of the department's leadership. This handbook is intended to provide essential information and strategies which will prove useful to both current and prospective leaders. Special emphasis is placed on the section dealing with the Chairman's role. This position is the linchpin in departmental progress. The handbook is not an operational manual but provides an overview of essential information.

TARGET AUDIENCE

The contents of the manual are directed principally to the leadership of departments, but they should also prove useful to all department staff members and administrators in the hospital environment. The discussion and recommendations included are generic so as to be useful to a broad spectrum of programs and institutions. The Handbook may also be used to introduce new Residents to hospital management and administrative practice.

Goal

The main goal is to prepare department leaders to manage their departments, in an effective and efficient manner, consistent with the mission of the institution. The format of this handbook includes some historical background on the development of hospitals, the evolution of hospital dentistry, issues of structure, governance, leadership and management. There is *no attempt to focus on clinical aspects of practice*. Current regulations and standards are considered in recommending practices.

HOSPITAL DEVELOPMENT

Hospitals reflect the level of civilization humanity has achieved and the degrees to which individuals care about one another. Their origins can be traced over many centuries to the establishment in India of what may have been the first hospital in the third century BC.

Hospitals have reached their greatest sophistication in the United States by serving first the poor and then the rich, throughout the development of institutional care. Today's hospitals are typically large, socially complex, public-oriented institutions that employ the most up-to-date and sophisticated technology. Throughout the evolution of hospitals their primary purposes have remained unchanged: "The primary function of the hospital, the one which has been constant throughout the whole of its evolution is to care for the sick and injured."

Hospitals have developed other important community functions, which, although subordinate to the primary purpose are recognized as part of the hospital's responsibility because they contribute to the care of the sick.

The variety of hospitals has proliferated: large and small, for profit and non-profit, teaching and non-teaching, privately owned and public, church and community owned, and special purpose. All, nevertheless, share a common mission—to care for the sick and injured.

HOSPITALS IN THE UNITED STATES

In the 1700's the seaport towns of Boston, Philadelphia, New York, Newport (Rhode Island), and Charleston (South Carolina) were among the most populous in the colonies. As these cities grew, so did the necessity for providing some level of refuge for shipboard victims of contagious diseases. Rest houses, isolation hospitals, and quarantine stations organized to segregate individuals with contagious diseases from the population at large, arose in response to this need. The following almshouses and hospitals were noted for the quality care they provided:

- Philadelphia Almshouse (circa 1713) an institution founded by William Penn and open only to Quakers

- Bellevue Hospital (1736) a descendant of the Poor House of the City of New York

- Charleston Almshouse (1738) a combination refuge for prisoners and paupers, serving mainly chronic cases Charity Hospital, New Orleans (1737), a hospital and an asylum for indigent people.

Hospitals moved west with the shifting population. Migration and population growth necessitated new types of hospitals classified according to population served and ownership status:

1. Nonprofit voluntary hospitals—These hospitals are usually categorized as follows:

   - Community sponsored

   - Church sponsored

   - Foundation sponsored

2. For-profit hospitals—These hospitals are sometimes referred to as proprietary hospitals and are broadly categorized as follows:

   - Privately owned, usually by physicians either individually or as a group corporate, or investor owned, as exemplified by the large chains

3. Public hospitals—These include city or county-owned and acute general care hospitals and state hospitals for the mentally ill

4. Federal government hospitals

   - Public health service hospitals

   - Veterans Administration medical centers

   - Armed forces (Army, Navy, Air Force) hospitals

Nonprofit voluntary hospitals are the oldest and most important links in the evolutionary chain. They have been on the cutting edge of changes that shaped the modern hospital. The following examples illustrate the importance of nonprofit voluntary hospitals to the growth and improvement of modern hospitals.

Pennsylvania Hospital in Philadelphia opened in 1752 and was the first permanent hospital established within the United States. Its charter authorized the hospital's contributors to make all laws and regulations relating to the hospital and required them to meet annually to elect a twelve-person board of managers. The board limited physician power, although in most cases it deferred to the judgment of competent physicians. The Pennsylvania Hospital's mission was to serve the "useful and laborious" poor rather than those who could work but refused.

New York Hospital was another important early hospital. Chartered in 1771, it was completed in 1775. Because of fire and military medical needs during the Revolutionary War, the first civilian patients were not admitted until 1791. New York Hospital's mission was to accommodate the sick poor. However, patients who were able to pay some portion of their expenses were expected to contribute. Patients who were able to pay but were also healthy enough to work donated their services: cleaning rooms, doing laundry and nursing others. A separate building housed patients with mental illness. New York Hospital received large grants from the State to finance construction and care for indigent patients.

Massachusetts General Hospital, another groundbreaking institution, was incorporated in 1811. Its focus on providing much needed hospital training to medical students in New England, distinguished Massachusetts General Hospital from the previous two mentioned hospitals.

Advances in science and medicine during the mid-nineteenth century greatly enriched hospitals, which then became important centers for disseminating knowledge, and places in which all classes of society could benefit from treatment. Improvements in eliminating or reducing pain and controlling sepsis transformed surgery and expanded the hospital's role in providing more human science-based treatment. During the nineteenth century, hospitals became involved with the medical school curriculum. Clinical methods established in hospitals enhanced research and promoted improved teaching.

New technology, increased knowledge and societal pressures led to changes in hospital roles over the decades. For example, as the germ theory of disease and aseptic techniques became better understood, the number of infections decreased. As a result the makeup of the patient population changed drastically as patients in all financial brackets became aware of the health advantages of being treated in hospitals.

Paying patient wards and expensive private rooms emerged, changing forever the method of financing hospitals. More recently, concerns about cost, efficiency and effectiveness have arisen in the hospital industry.

As hospitals proliferated and operational costs skyrocketed, hospital revenue consumption grew at a rate the public could not support. The need for practical responses to managed care and concerns about rising costs led hospitals to assume many corporate characteristics and become more management centered.

The current corporate stage is characterized by emphasis on quality, consumer satisfaction, prudent and progressive fiscal management, and increased marketing activities. It requires a somewhat different pattern of behavior by all parties. It does not require change in fundamental social values.

Hospitals in the United States evolved through the following four stages

Stage 1: Refuge
  Board centered

Stage 2: Physician workshop
  Physician centered

Stage 3: Business
  Management centered

Stage 4: Corporate
  Polycentric

Historically the association of dentistry with hospitals is generally less well documented than is medical care. The reason being that the hospital is not the natural workshop for dentists and for many decades dentistry has played a peripheral role. There are, nonetheless, some significant dates in the development of "hospital dentistry".

The first known relationship of dentistry with hospitals in this country occurred in 1791 when an English immigrant dentist named Richard Skinner joined the staff of the New York Dispensary in New York City. In 1850 a dentist opened the Wheeling Hospital (West VA) "to treat a variety of problems beyond oral problems". In 1869 Dr. James Garretson, an oral surgeon, was appointed to the staff of the University of Pennsylvania Hospital in Philadelphia. The first dental intern (Resident) was appointed in Philadelphia in the year 1901 at the Philadelphia General Hospital. In 1944, the American Dental Association appointed a special committee on Hospital Dental Services. This committee was succeeded in 1948 by the Council at Hospital Dental Services.

In 1960 a Commission by the American Council of Education included the following recommendation:

> "If dentistry is to perform its central function of providing dental health care to American people it cannot continue to be centered solely around the office and the laboratory. The commission believes it feasible and desirable that dentists participate in total health care by serving on the staffs of hospital, with status consistent with that of practitioners of other health professions".

Additional significant dates relating to the development of the accreditation process may be found in Appendix I.

PUBLIC NEEDS AND INTERESTS

The public has come to rely on the hospital as the place where the indigent, low income and medically complicated seek high quality care. It is the location where the indigent can achieve access to "cutting-edge" technology and evidence based care. In the current economic environment however, this pattern of utilization, which includes substantial numbers of indigent patients, poses problems for hospitals and funders alike. This fact is sometimes the source of misunderstanding and conflict between administration and clinical staff, as each side sees its responsibilities differently.

HOSPITAL NEEDS AND INTERESTS

Hospital care is constantly changing in response to new information, new diseases and new technology. Hospitals are therefore not limited to the care of the indigent; instead, they treat individuals requiring special attention available only in the confines of the hospital. They provide specialty care and utilize high technology equipment.

In addition to attempting to provide the highest quality of care, hospitals are interested in enhancing their reputations, so as to obtain a competitive edge and increasing their marketability. Clinicians are partners in this effort.

EDUCATION

Dental departments with Residency Programs, usually, are established in teaching hospitals but may also be found in community general hospitals. Residency programs in general have the beneficial effect of attracting qualified faculty and producing well-trained residents. Some hospitals also accommodate other educational programs.

One study for instance, conducted in New York several years ago, identified 1,460 students from twenty-three schools (other than dental school,) who were training in hospitals. A large variety of programs which required dental infrastructure for training and education were supported in the New York City municipal system. Dental departments also conduct basic clinical research.

There are two main philosophies which underlie general dentistry residency programs. Some others view them as remedial programs conducted as an extension of pre-doctoral education transitional programs which provide additional advanced preparation for subsequent practice. Although training programs generally benefit hospitals, not all hospitals (for a variety of reasons), are in a position to take advantage of their benefits. The Council on Dental Accreditation (CODA) through its Standards and Guidelines requires the transitional program.

PROFESSIONAL DEVELOPMENT

The Hospital environment encourages a high level of professionalism on the part of the dental staff. There exists the opportunity to function as a team member with many other health care disciplines and specialties. Attendance at conferences and grand rounds, collaboration with multi-specialty and inter-disciplinary colleagues is made easier, and the opportunity to care for a broad spectrum of medically complex individuals is an important societal contribution. The consultation system, which is an important element of hospital practice, is also a potential source of practice growth, education and collaboration.

SECTION II

HOSPITAL STRUCTURE AND GOVERNANCE

Section 2

STRUCTURE

The hospital is one of the most complex organizations in society, a microcosm of the wider society.

Hospital organization comprises a mix of internal systems and subsystems that interact with the external environment in a manner that reduces waste, eliminates inefficiency and most importantly, promotes quality of care.

In order to effectively carry out their role, most hospitals establish an organizational model encompassing five major areas. They are:

1. Finance

2. Operations

3. Plant Maintenance

4. Medical Care

5. Human Relations

GOVERNANCE

Hospitals are usually administered by a governing board called The Board of Trustees, Board of Directors, or other similar title in compliance with state laws which require all established corporate entities to have a board.

The Board also has three major functions:

- They control and maintain organizational effectiveness

- They help obtain support for the hospital from its environment

- They represent the community as a whole and sub-groups within the community to which they are accountable.

The Board also sets policies under which both medical and administrative procedures are developed, and it has final responsibility for the following:

- Quality of medical care provided in the hospital

- Appointment of medical staff members

- Appointment of the hospital administrator, or ChiefExecutive Officer (CEO), who is responsible for daily operations

- Services provided by the hospital

- Protection of investments in the hospital

- Prudent use of assets and income

The Board meets regularly to receive reports from which it formulates and modifies policies and actions. It keeps abreast of changing health-care patterns and their effects on the community. The Board is responsible for the ultimate financial and legal affairs of the corporation (hospitals). Their policies limit and constrain management's operational decision-making, choice and action.

ORGANIZATION

In order to achieve its mission, the staff of the hospital is grouped according to responsibilities. This results in the display of the well-known Table of Organization (TO). The Table of Organization varies in complexity according to institutional size. In the past TOs have been hierarchical in form and vertical in appearance. More recent functional TOs tend to be more horizontal, reflecting staffing patterns that are more team oriented. Current hospital organization reflects not only the peculiar needs of hospitals but also embodies fundamental principles of corporate organization. Tables of Organization—a collection of boxes and lines are used to group related functions and satisfy management principles of efficiency, accountability, control and coordination. They are designed to define a reasonable span of control, and improve communication.

Line administrators supervise activities contributing directly to the products (health care) of the institution. Staff administrators contribute indirectly by providing services or advice to the line organization. Both line and staff administrators facilitate functions such as coordination and communication, maintaining an acceptable span of control and a short chain of command.

LEGAL ISSUES

The governing body of all health care institutions has three main functions:

1. To develop short- and long-range institutional goals

2. To appoint staff to senior administrative and medical positions

3. To evaluate the professional performance of administrators and medical staff

Moreover in the new corporate culture, the governing body has become more heavily involved in the following aspects of information management:

- Public relations

- Community relations

- Marketing

- Fund-raising

- Finance

The Board must also ensure that its organization and that of the administration and medical staff are appropriate to carry out all responsibilities. For example, the board must be sure that its Executive Committee functions properly in executing board policy between meetings of the full board. The Executive Committee cannot usurp the prerogatives of the board to make extraordinary decisions, nor should it be permitted independently to delegate group responsibilities to any individual member of the committee.

Typical hospital board committees include the following:

- Finance

- Buildings, Grounds and Capital

- Personnel

- Public relations

- Education

- Medical advisory (sometimes called Professional Affairs or Joint Conference committee)

Each committee deals with specific responsibilities as assigned and makes recommendations to the full governing board. Committee structure and administration are governed by the corporate bylaws, which are themselves defined by state incorporation statutes. These bylaws and statutes define the powers, duties, and limitations of all hospital committees. Bylaws, rules, regulations, and all subsequent amendments must be approved by the Board of Trustees. The Board of

Trustees is legally responsible for all activities and accountable to the public for the conduct of the institution.

ADMINISTRATION

The organizational structure of hospitals is tri-partite. A triad determines the activities of the hospital. The three members of the triad are:

- The Governing Board
- The Administration
- The Medical Staff

Operational management of the hospital rests with the President or CEO. The corporate phase of hospital development (previously described), is characterized by a heightened concern for the patient (customer) and by increased corporate competition. These factors, over time, have led to the vertical integration of a broad spectrum of health care and social services. Examples of services provided by a single institution are:

- Ambulatory services
- Acute general care services
- Long-term care services
- Wellness Services

Many corporate entities have become pivotal institutions in health-care systems by combining the above-mentioned services into a single integrated system.

The challenge for the dental director in such an arrangement lies in devising a system for providing high-quality training for residents and care for all patients in such systems.

Patient Support Areas [Administrative]

Patient support areas include Admitting, Food Service and Nutrition, Hospital Safety and Security, Social Services, Chaplaincy, Patient Representative and Community Relations.

ADMITTING

Support services are subdivided into medical and patient support services and administrative support services. A tiered organizational structure has evolved to ensure competent performance of these support services. (See below).

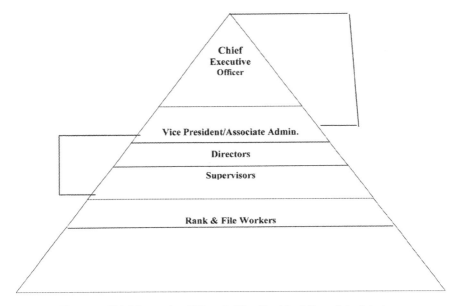

Diagram: Chief Executive Officer & Vice President/Associate Admin. =
Corporate Staff
Supervisors & Rank & File Workers = Supervisory Staff

Medical staff organizational structure also reflects the hierarchical structure of the hospital. The Chief Medical Officer is guided by a medical executive committee and several standing committees which conduct business as assigned.

The Admitting Department receives and registers all patients who use the hospital services. Data collected during these processes are vital to the quality of care and financial health of the hospital. This department combines duties involving public relations, business procedures and clinical matters. The first impression of the hospital is often formed from contact with this department. They also conduct pre-admission screening, inpatient registration, patient placement and census management.

FOOD SERVICE AND NUTRITION (DIETARY)

This department prepares food for both patients and employees. It utilizes 6%–10% of the hospital's workforce. The food service operation can be affected by shortened lengths of stay, profit incentives, degree of computerization and the increased emphasis on good nutrition. In some instances, they may also operate a coffee shop as well as prepare specialized meals.

HOSPITAL SAFETY AND SECURITY

Hospital security may be defined as a system of safeguards designed to protect the physical property of the facility and achieve relative safety for all people interacting within the hospital. Security is intended to reduce the number of detrimental incidents occurring within the hospital environment. Hospital safety and security are not law enforcement functions but instead operate under limits set by the institution.

Hospital security embodies many aspects peculiar to the institutional setting. For example, the facility remains open and therefore must be secure 24 hours a day. The sick and injured must have access at any time, and the activities of visitors and the business operations of gift shops, pharmacies, cashiers, physicians' offices, and others must not be unduly hindered. All entrances and exits must be covered or videoed. Because patients ultimately pay the bills, their security needs also are considered within the organizational framework.

SOCIAL SERVICES

Hospital-based medical social services date back to 1905. These services resulted from the realization of the value of having a professional help patients and families with problems caused by social conditions. The role of social workers in hospitals has expanded significantly since 1905 and continues to evolve as the institutional delivery of medical care becomes more complicated.

Today's medical social worker improves the effectiveness of the hospital by assisting the patient in solving personal social problems related to family relationships, employment, finances, and legal issues. Physical discomfort, isolation, fear, and anxiety are all areas contributing to the illness itself or interfering with treatment.

Social Services department functions fall within three broad categories:

1. Service to the hospital

2. Service to the patient

3. Service to the community

The most significant of these functions is service to patients and families, which includes the following tasks:

- Planning discharge from the hospital
- Screening and case finding for at-risk populations
- Providing psychosocial assessments
- Counseling patients and family members
- Assisting patients with financial arrangements
- Providing information about community services and benefits
- Making referrals to other sources

As a result of the growth of managed care, prospective payment systems and the emphasis on shortening length of stay, the social worker is playing a larger role in managing length of stay by facilitating the discharge of patients.

CHAPLAINCY

The American Hospital Association's *Manual on Hospital Chaplaincy* states the important role chaplains play within the hospital:

> The American Hospital Association recognizes that chaplaincy programs are a necessary part of the hospital's provision for total patient care, and that qualified chaplains and adequate facilities, as well as the support of administration and medical staff, are essential in carrying out an effective ministry of patients.

The chaplain is an essential member of the health-care team. Chaplains often deal with diverse concerns such as the patient's and family's anxiety, the economics of illness, and the increasing number of health-care personnel with whom the patient interacts.

The chaplain performs several pastoral functions:

- Assisting the patient's orientation to institutional life
- Representing the patient's religious community and expressing its concern and care
- Making known the religious services available within the institution

In many hospitals, chaplains are required to see each new patient. Several categories of patients command the special attention of pastoral care. They include the following:

- Patients going into surgery
- Patients who are dangerously and critically ill
- Patients who have long-term illnesses
- Patients in the maternity ward
- Children
- Patients who are mentally ill
- Patients who are terminally ill

PATIENT REPRESENTATIVE

The role of the patient representative has grown over the years as patients' rights concerns have become more prominent in hospitals. The Joint Commission on Accreditation of Healthcare Organization (JCAHO) has devoted a section of its standards to patients' rights and organizational ethics. The preamble to this section states the following: the goal of this function is to recognize and respect each patient in the provision of care in accord with the fundamental human, civil constitutional and statutory rights to improve patient outcome.

Medical Records Department

The Medical Records Department is arguably one of the most important administrative departments. Its importance is reflected by the fact that in most hospitals there is a medical records committee with representation from both the medical staff and administration. It is the lifeblood of the institution with the central responsibility for collecting and processing most important data in the institution. The medical records department maintains the history of each patient's experience from admission to discharge. It does this in a manner which complies with the standards set by the regulatory agencies and the guidelines of the institution.

The information maintained by medical records department is also used as a basis in legal actions and quality assurance reviews. Included in the department's responsibility are data used for planning purposes, clinical data and statistical data. The department's information is a broad based indicator of patient's care which is useful to:

- Patients
- Doctors
- Hospital administrators
- Teachers
- Students
- Researchers
- National and international agencies

SECTION III

MEDICAL/DENTAL STAFF

Section 3

CHAIRPERSON/DIRECTOR ROLE

The basic *role* of the chairperson or director is prescribed in the by-Laws of the institution and the *responsibilities* by job description (see appendix 1). The Chairperson is the "boss" responsible for the administration of the department, the training of residents and any other educational activities that may take place within the department. The chairperson is also responsible for assisting in the medical administration of the institution through service on committees and other interactions with colleagues.

Possibly the most important role for a dental director, however, does not appear in any formal position description. That role is *leadership*: a role which is defined in many different ways by different authors. It is, by my own definition an imprecise pattern of behavior—more art than science, which results in the achievement of desired results in implementing a mission.

Dental departments for many decades have had a peripheral status in hospitals. As notions of comprehensive primary care have evolved, the role of the importance of dentistry in hospitals, has changed from a singular focus on surgical procedures to greater emphasis on comprehensive general dentistry including all specialties. As a result dental departments in general have emerged as autonomous departments, no longer a section or division of the Department of General Surgery.

This section deals with the role of chairperson as leader (external actions) and less so with the responsibility of chairperson as boss (internal control), although the two are not mutually exclusive. Internal responsibilities will be discussed later in this document. The essential elements of effective leadership include strong management skills, the ability to influence others, good communication skills, personal integrity, ethical conduct and self confidence. As dentistry has attained full departmental status in the hospital setting, it is essential that its leadership possesses the above characteristics. The chairperson must be professional, provide clear direction, possess the ability to motivate and implement and to navigate the complex hospital environment.

To quote Margaret Wheatley (renowned leadership futurist and organizational development expert), **"In organizations, real power and energy are generated through relationships. The patterns of relationships and the**

capacities to form them are more important than tasks, functions, roles and positions."

This quotation is especially appropriate as dental departments find themselves in the competitive environment both within the institution and outside. This situation is brought about by the attainment of full department status. The leader must create a favorable environment through challenging, but realistic goal setting, establishing performance standards and advocacy on behalf of the department.

The ability to understand the environment at all times and gauge the climate at other specific times is critical to success. It is worth emphasizing the importance of clear, lucid and complete communication (both upwards and downwards) as essential in providing good leadership. Many institutions which sponsor residency programs have created two separate leadership positions; namely, Chairperson and Program Director. Where this arrangement exists there is the opportunity for sharing the workload of growing and managing the department.

The key to maximizing this organizational arrangement often lies with the Chair's willingness and ability to delegate responsibility.

It provides the opportunity for the chairperson to devote his/her time to those external relationships which benefit the department. (See Appendix 1)

The Program Director has primary responsibility for those functions prescribed in the Commission On Dental Accreditation standards. (see Appendix 2)

LEADERSHIP

(Leader vs Boss)

Dental departments tend to employ small staffs who perform specialized functions. Small staffs present the important advantage of manageability.

Sometimes small staffs also create the disadvantage of functional gaps. One frequently observed gap is the absence or failure of marketing activity. The chairperson must therefore assume broad responsibility for that important but often overlooked function of marketing the department, both internally within the hospital and externally in the community at large.

The internal marketing of departmental services increases the value of the department within the institution as well as enhances its integration. The opportunity for sharing in the educational burden and in the referral patterns is expanded by visible and substantive contributions to its broader activities. External marketing, aimed at consumers, creates increased opportunities for service and for furthering the mission of the institution. In the current competitive climate, considerably more time than is customary should be devoted to seeking external support and independent funding.

STRATEGIC PLANNING

Strategic planning is an essential element of the leadership function. It is however not without its challenges. It is time consuming; it requires flexibility, and sometimes nimbleness. It is an interactive process which requires a level of internal scrutiny which may expose uncomfortable weaknesses within a department.

Strategic Planning (SP) is an essential leadership tool. It is closely associated with the attribute of "Creativity". Creativity and innovation contribute to establishing a **Vision** for the department. SP creates an institutional and departmental early preparation system for anticipated changes. It is a means of coping with accelerating changes in the environment. The earlier that changes are anticipated, the more time will be available for preparation to meet those challenges.

Among many definitions of strategic planning is the one which states that *"Strategic Planning is the science and art of deploying all the resources of the business (personnel, materials, money and management) in achieving established goals and objectives successfully in the face of competition". (John D. Glover and Gerald A Simon) Strategic thinking is the essence of strategic planning. It is the process of creating a vision for the department and charting a strategic course of action to make that vision a reality. Strategic Planning is not the process of predicting the future nor is it management of the operation. It involves making reasonable assumptions to project outcomes under prudent risks.*

Boss of the operation on the other hand is concerned with day-to-day issues such as hiring and firing, inventory control and appointment systems, etc. They fall under the "boss role". Strategic Planning on the other hand is clearly a leadership function, an ongoing process that is future oriented. Strategic planning is more a political and negotiating process than a quantitative exercise. Therefore, the success of the process depends not only on the formulation of the strategies but also, and more importantly, on integrating it into the daily management of the activities.

Leadership styles vary across a broad spectrum. They range from an autocratic style at one end, which reflects a high degree of management control to the other end where there is a free-rein style reflecting a higher degree of employee or staff control. In between there are paternalistic, participative and delegative styles of leadership. Regardless of the style adopted, there exists certain core principles, which are common to all styles.

The United States Army Handbook (1973) for instance lists eleven principles which define leadership style.

1. Know yourself (*constantly seek self improvement*)

2. Be technically proficient (*as a leader*)

3. Seek and take responsibility

4. Make sound and timely decisions

5. Set the example

6. Know and care for your workers

7. Keep your workers informed

8. Develop a sense of responsibility in your workers

9. Ensure that tasks are understood, supervised and accomplished.
    (Clear, explicit, detailed communication and reasonable task assignments are important to this responsibility.)

10. Train as a team

11. Use the full capabilities of your organization (*department, section*)

The effective leader selects and trains staff carefully, trusts completely and creates opportunities for them to grow and perform. Effectiveness is enhanced by skill in delegation as distinct from the art of supervision. True delegation can sometimes prove difficult for leaders who are wedded to the practice of supervision (the close monitoring of relatively small tasks). Delegation in contrast to supervision refers to the transfer of responsibilities for a substantive part of the operation. Skillful delegation can be a source of creativity, "state-of-the-art" information, new ideas and renewed energy.

PROCESS OF LEADERSHIP

The process of leadership is so important and critical to success that the JCAHO has itself included a separate standard in its manual covering the topic. Its concepts are worth inclusion since their description is specific to the health care sector.

As enunciated by JCAHO, leadership requires the competent performance of the following four processes (Figure 2-1):

1. Planning services—leaders create a mission statement reflecting long-range, short-range, strategic and operational plans; resource allocation; and organizational policies.

2. Directing services—Leaders organize, direct and staff patient care and support services according to the scope and requirements of services offered.

3. Implementing and coordinating services—Leaders integrate patient care and support services throughout the organizations.

4. Improving services—leaders establish expectations and plans and manage processes to measure, assess, and improve the performance of the organization's governance, management clinical and support processes. [See figure below]

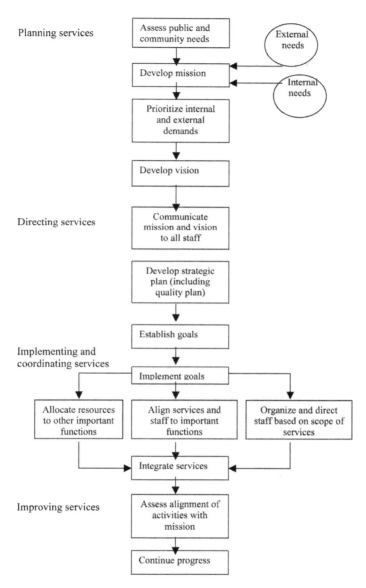

Planning services

Assess public and community needs

External needs

Develop mission

Internal needs

Prioritize internal and external demands

Develop vision

Directing services

Communicate mission and vision to all staff

Develop strategic plan (including quality plan)

Establish goals

Implementing and coordinating services

Implement goals

Allocate resources to other important functions

Align services and staff to important functions

Organize and direct staff based on scope of services

Integrate services

Improving services

Assess alignment of activities with mission

Continue progress

Leadership function. (From Joint Commission on Accreditation of Healthcare Organizations: (*Comprehensive accreditation manual for hospitals, Chicago, 1995, The Commission.*)

The Process

The Strategic Planning process requires six key steps—external environmental analysis, internal program and organizational analysis SWOT (strengths, weaknesses, opportunity, threat) analysis, definition of program mission, evaluation of strategic issues and options and definition of strategic action plans.

The following table provides a framework for analysis:

FRAMEWORK FOR STRATEGIC ANALYSIS

ENVIRONMENT	DEPARTMENT	PEOPLE
Market Demand	Key Characteristics	Leadership
Need/Demand	Department Strengths & Weaknesses	
Technology	Capital vs. labor Intensive	Vision
Level of Investment	Staffing	
Competition	Product Definition	Generalist skills
Institution & Private Sector	Program Strengths	Staffing
Government	Who is the customer	
Patient Support, Regulations, Funding	Payor source	

Implementation of the analytic process must include the definition of specific goals which encompass the desired long-term achievements. It must also specify *quantifiable* objectives which support the goals and which establish a specific timeframe for their completion. Key personnel and stakeholders must also be involved in the process. Failure to follow any of the steps will result in a deficient, diminished, or failed plan.

MEDICAL/DENTAL STAFF

Many hospitals refer to their clinical staffs as the medical/dental staff giving evidence to the important status of dental programs in those hospitals.

The medical/dental staffs are responsible for both patient care and for providing professional leadership of the organization. They are expected to provide clinically appropriate and scientifically valid care of the highest standards.

They are also expected to participate in assessment of both clinical and non-clinical processes which contribute to the quality of patient care.

Medical staff organization and governance are usually delineated in the hospital by-laws. By-laws is the instrument which prescribes staff membership, the credentialing process and the committee structures necessary for implementing activities of the institution.

By-laws are also usually accompanied by a set of rules and regulations which frame the operational limits of the medical/dental staff. They must be approved by the governing body before they become effective.

Writing and approval of the By-Laws is a major activity of the medical staff. They require approval both by the Medical Executive Committee and the governing board in order to amend them. A bylaws committee is often appointed to draft them.

By-laws should be available and required reading for all clinical staff since they cover the following important elements:

- Composition of Medical Executive Committee
- Due process mechanisms for medical staff
- Corrective actions
- Complete description of the medical staff organization including rank and officers

The bylaws also regulate the following:

1. The method of selecting officers
2. The qualifications, responsibilities and tenure of officers
3. The conditions and mechanisms for removing officers from their positions
4. Requirements for frequency of meetings and for attendance

5. Mechanisms designed to facilitate effective communication among the medical staff, hospital administration and the governing body

In those hospitals sponsoring or participating in professional graduate education programs, the rules, regulations and policies specify the mechanisms by which house staff members are supervised by medical staff members in carrying out their patient care responsibilities.

In hospitals with many levels of governance, mechanisms are established to allow the medical staff to communicate with all individuals and departments involved in policy decisions affecting patient care. The bylaws provide procedures for both their adoption and amendment and reflect the hospital's current practices concerning medical staff organization and functions.

By-laws are presented in the form of a series of Articles. Each Article covers an important group of topics. For example, a typical Table of Contents would look somewhat like the following:

CONTENTS

Preamble

Article I	Definitions
Article II	Membership
Article III	Categories of Medical Staff
Article IV	Allied Health Clinicians
Article V	Appointment Process
Article VI	Temporary Privileges
Article VII	Reappointment Changes in Clinical Privileges and continuation or Supervision of Clinical Privileges
Article VIII	Hearing and Appeal Procedures
Article IX	Organization of Medical Staff
Article X	Clinical Objectives
Article XI	Committees
Article XII	Amendments

The bylaws are usually accompanied by another document, entitled Rules and Regulations, which provide a framework for implementation of the bylaws. Rules and regulations are not limited to clinical practice but include systems at the interface of clinical, administrative and support systems. They are presented in sections.

A typical list of sections would look like the following:

Section I	Staff Dues/Assessments Penalties
Section II	Admissions/General Care/Discharge
Section III	Medical Records
Section IV	Drug Orders and Order-Writing Procedures
Section V	Patient Rights and Consent
Section VI	Consultations
Section VII	Disaster Plan
Section VIII	Billing
Section IX	Types of Patients
Section X	Continuing Medical Education
Section XI	Professional Liability Coverage
Section XII	Adoption and Amendment

APPOINTMENT/CREDENTIALING

The credentialing and appointment processes are especially important to the Director of the Dental Department. It is a serious responsibility of the Director who, in carrying out these functions, is acting on behalf of the Board of Trustees since only the Board is legally authorized to make appointments to the Medical Staff.

The appointment process is designed to assure that all applicants are screened and evaluated carefully prior to presentation to the Board of Trustees. The process can be initiated either verbally or in writing from the practitioner or from the department's chairperson.

The formal application must include at least detailed information concerning:

- Current licensure and registration
- Professional education and training

- Current competence (documenting a continuing ability to provide patient care services at an acceptable level of quality and efficiency)

- Cooperativeness—ability to work with other providers both clinically and administratively

- Satisfaction of membership obligations, i.e., compliance with basic obligations in the several articles of the bylaws

- Professional Ethics and Conduct—to be of good moral character and adhere to generally recognized standards of professional ethics

Subsequent to the submission of the application, the next step in the appointment process is verification of all information. This step is followed by review by the Credentials Committee of the Medical Board. This Committee reviews the application and, in addition to certifying the accuracy of the information, they examine the applicant's legal liability status, discuss the details of current or past malpractice cases, and ascertain the presence of appropriate professional liability insurance coverage. The Credentials Committee will also assure that:

- The applicant is free from mental or physical impairment which would prevent the performance of his/her duties

- The applicant is free from substance abuse practice

- The applicant possesses the requisite verbal and communication skills

- Verification of hospital and community need

The applicant may be required to appear in person to be interviewed by the Credentials Committee and to present the requisite documentation in its original form.

APPOINTMENT CATEGORIES

After the successful conclusion of the credentialing process, the committee forwards its recommendation to the medical board. The medical board in turn forwards its recommendation to the Board of Trustees for its action. Completion of this process will result in appointment to one of four main categories of staff.

The usual categories are:

1. Active Staff—the staff, which provides the bulk of clinical Services, because of privileges which permit them to admit and care for patients.

They may also hold office and vote on board committees. Most hospitals establish a hierarchical system among attending staff. The usual pattern is Assistant Attending, Associate Attending and Attending in ascending order. The level of appointment is based on professional attainment.

2. Courtesy Staff—They may admit and treat patients and exercise clinical privileges, subject to specific limitations of the bylaws. They may neither hold offices nor vote.

3. Consulting Staff—Comprising highly qualified non-voting members of the medical staff who by virtue of their expertise are permitted to advise the active staff on matters of patient care.

4. Honorary Staff—Members of this group are individuals who have served the specialty with distinction and have retired from active clinical practice. They may not hold office, vote, nor admit patients

After the appropriate category has been determined, clinical privileges are recommended by the chairperson and they become effective after approval by the medical executive committee. Privileges are certified by a document entitled "Delineation of Privileges"; one copy of which is retained in the appointee's personal file. The approval of privileges is based on a careful review of the applicant's training, experience and track record. It has the legal force of defining the scope of practice and the approval by signature of the chairperson is required.

Some hospitals define other additional staff categories in their Bylaws such as:

Affiliated Staff

This group consists of physicians and dentists in the community who meet general requirements and desire to refer patients to the hospital for inpatient care, specialized or outpatient care, and still maintain contact with their patients. They are not permitted to exercise the privilege of an attending staff member such as admitting patients, writing notes or orders. They may, however, access their patients' medical records and visit their patients.

Other Health Professionals

These are health care professionals who are licensed to practice their professions. They comprise two groups—(1) Independent Other Health Professionals who do not require physician or dentist supervision and (2) Dependent Other Health

Professionals who are licensed staff members. Their services are performed under the supervision of a responsible staff member.

TEMPORARY PRIVILEGES

Temporary privileges to admit and treat patients are sometimes granted, on the basis of demonstrated need. The applicant is required to submit the same documentation as if applying for permanent appointment to the staff. An expedited process is followed along the lines required for permanent appointment. These privileges are often approved by the chairman of the Medical Executive Committee directly.

COMMITTEES

Those functions of the medical staff not performed by staff officers or carried out by the members at general meetings of the staff, shall be performed by committees and subcommittees of the staff. Bylaws establish Standing Committees which are those committees mandated either by external agencies or by customary hospital practice and are required for operation of the hospital. They meet on a regularly scheduled basis to conduct the business of the hospital. They each have a predetermined agenda. The complexity of hospital management over time has required the formation of a system of subcommittees to distribute the workload and take advantage of available experience and expertise. The bylaws are designed to organize the complexity into more manageable systems that can be implemented. A representative list of committees and subcommittees would look like the following:

Standing Committees and Subcommittees

    A.   Executive Medical Board

    B.   Credentials Committee

        i. Subcommittee for credentialing of Other Health Care Professionals

    C.   Bylaws Committee

    D.   Utilization Management Committee

E. Specialized Care Committee, with the following standing subcommittees:

   i. Operating Room Subcommittee

   ii. Trauma Subcommittee

   iii. Critical Care Subcommittee

   iv. Emergency Care Subcommittee

   v. Cancer Coordinating Subcommittee

   vi. Laser Safety Subcommittee

F. Professional Conduct Committee, with the following standing subcommittees:

   i. Ethics, Education and Consultation Subcommittee

   ii. Surgical Care Review Subcommittee

   iii. Blood Utilization Subcommittee

G. Hospital Services Subcommittee

H. Pharmacy, Therapeutics and Nutrition Committee, with the following standing Subcommittees:

   i. Pharmacy and Therapeutics Subcommittee

   ii. Nutrition Subcommittee

I. Infection Surveillance Committee, with the following standing subcommittees:

   i. Infection Control Subcommittee

   ii. AIDS Subcommittee

J. Special Committees and Subcommittees

   i. Graduate Medical Education Committee

   ii. Radiation Safety Committee

   iii. Protection of Human Subjects Subcommittee

   iv. Quality Improvement Committee

   v. Ethics Committee

    vi. Research Committee

Appointment to membership on committees and subcommittees is prescribed in the bylaws. In most institutions, a two-year term with provisions for renewal of appointment is the usual practice.

CLINICAL SERVICES

The medical/dental staff is organized around clinical services. Each clinical service functions as a unit for the maintenance, evaluation, and improvement of patient care provided by that service. These objectives are attained through ongoing monitoring of patient care activities, conducting monthly assessment and evaluation activities, and implementing appropriate academic programs.

Examples of clinical services are:

1. Anesthesiology

2. Community and Preventive Medicine

3. Dental Medicine and Oral and Maxillofacial Surgery

4. Dermatology

5. Emergency Medicine

6. Family Medicine

7. Neurology

8. Neurosurgery

9. Obstetrics and Gynecology

10. Orthopedic Surgery

11. Ophthalmology

12. Pathology and Laboratory Medicine

13. Pediatrics

14. Podiatry

15. Psychiatry

16. Radiological Sciences

17. Radiation Oncology

18. Surgery

19. Thoracic Surgery

In most cases clinical services will depend on size, and type of hospital and community needs. Clinical services may be organized into departments, divisions or sections as directed in the bylaws. Hierarchically the department is the top controlling unit in a given service. The Department may subdivide into divisions and sections. The chairperson is responsible for organization of the clinical service. This responsibility includes appointments and reappointments of staff, setting clinical practice standards, professional ethics, and all matters relevant to clinical performance in accordance with the bylaws, rules and regulations.

The Chairperson is also the chief academic and administrative officer of the department. The Chair has the authority and responsibility to administer the service in accordance with the bylaws.

DUTIES OF THE CHAIRPERSON

The specific duties of the Chair include:

- Plan, develop, implement and supervise the activities of the department
- Develop, submit and administer the department's budget
- Conduct meetings and appoint committees as needed
- Assign tasks
- Evaluate staff performance and review all professional performances

In the current health care environment, the chairperson of a dental department should also devote considerable time to seeking external financial support such as grants, research funding and corporate support. He/She must provide leadership in taking advantage of current and emerging technology for educational, management and research purposes. The dental chairperson should be a good boss, an effective team leader, informed liaison, a knowledgeable communicator and an effective coordinator.

SECTIONS

Sections are even a smaller subdivisions of a department which focuses its activities on a more sharply focused set of activities, usually those of a subspecialty. Chiefs of Sections are responsible to the department chair, but they may report through a division chief depending on the individual hospital arrangement.

THE EXECUTIVE COMMITTEE

The Executive Committee (EC) is the preeminent committee of the medical staff. It serves as the conduit for information and actions between the staff, the Administration and the Governance. It is the principal committee responsible for formulating medical policy.

The EC's main responsibilities are as follows:

1. Responsible for making recommendations to the Board of Governors through the appropriate channels.

2. Receive and act on reports and recommendations from all standing and special committees of the Staff, the Hospital clinical departments and any other assigned activity groups.

3. Represent and act on behalf of the staff on all matters arising between meetings of the staff.

4. Coordinate the activities and general policies of the various clinical services of the hospital.

5. Develop clinical standards and policies.

6. Provide liaison among the staff, the CEO and the board.

7. Take the necessary steps to implement and enforce the hospital and staff Bylaws, Policies, Rules and Regulations.

8. Review the depth, scope and quality of the clinical services of the hospital.

9. Be accountable to the Board of Trustees, as representatives of the staff, for the medical care rendered to patients of the hospital.

10. Develop and transmit to the Joint Conference Committee, recommendations with respect to issues of hospital policy and provide interpretation of existing policies and regulations relating to patient care.

11. Provide advice and consultation to the Board of Trustees and to the administration, upon request.

12. Provide a mechanism for a fair and impartial hearing on matters of a disciplinary nature.

13. Form such committees as it deems necessary for consideration of matters pertaining to patient care, research, planning and other matters relative to the functioning of the Staff or the quality of patient care within the hospital.

SECTION IV

THE DENTAL DEPARTMENT

Section 4

The Dental Department

The Department of Dentistry's evolution in the hospital parallels the changing role of the hospital itself. For decades dental services or departments were peripheral to the mainstream of the hospital services and were therefore placed organizationally as part of the Department of Surgery.

Federal legislation passed in the 1960's made more funds available for health-care services. Medicare (Title 18) provided new funds for training programs as well as treatment programs. Medicaid (Title, 19) Office of Economic Opportunity (OEO) legislation, Comprehensive care, Regional Medical Plan, and other antipoverty legislation funded expansion of services and fueled demand for services including dental services.

At the same time the role of hospitals has changed so that they have become centers of health-care services. They now provide comprehensive ambulatory care services. It is within this environment that full service dental departments were established in many hospitals. In some institutions, services were expanded beyond oral surgery. Dentistry still remained a section within the Department of Surgery in many hospitals.

Subsequent to the 1960's, the American Dental Association's interest in hospital dentistry appears to have increased and the Council on Dental Accreditation (CODA) has instituted an accreditation process based on standards developed by the Council. In the late 1970's dentistry also obtained a seat on the Joint Commission on Accreditation of Health Care Organizations (JCAHO), a further step in recognition of dentistry's institutional role. These actions have contributed to the expansion of dentistry in the hospital setting.

One aim of a full service (training and service) dental department should be attainment of equal administrative status with other major departments within the hospital. For example, equal status with the departments of medicine and surgery should be the goal. This status must be reflected within the institution's official Table of Organizations.

The tendency to assign dentistry a different niche from the major departments still exists. It is not uncommon in a number of institutions to find the dental department reporting to the Chairman of Surgery or the Director of Ambulatory Care. Such arrangements inhibit the capacity of the dental department to achieve its full potential. Reporting to the Director of Ambulatory Care is especially inappropriate.

In the words of Paul Van Ostenberg, "The relationship of the dental department to management structure of the hospital will largely determine the flow of resources and information." Being perceived as a lower-tiered unit places the leadership at a disadvantage in key policy, and budgetary decision making. Direct access to the principal decision makers, especially those in Finance, Operations and Medical Policy is key to maximizing effectiveness.

The departmental Table of Organization (TO) should reflect the reality of the operation. Because dental department staffs are usually relatively small with roles that are well defined, the construction of the department's TO should be reasonably straightforward.

The TO nonetheless, should avoid the pitfalls created by expedient and inappropriate planning, violations of accepted norms and excessive reliance on personal relationships.

The goals of departmental organization should include:

- Improvement of operational efficiencies

- Improvement in information management including visibility and access

- Improvement in data accuracy to aid in regulatory compliance

- Improvement in organizational planning

Careful thought must be given to defining roles so as to prevent either wasteful duplication or staff conflict. There must be clarity in the assignment of staff responsibilities while still preserving the team approach.

RELATIONSHIP TO ADMINISTRATION

Two key components contribute to departmental success. First: in the perceived value of dentistry to the hospital and second: the inter-relationship (sometimes personal) between the dental department's leadership and the senior administration staff. Development of the components is clearly an important function of the chairperson.

The Dental Department's value to the institution is based on the following:

- Enhancement of the reputation of the institution due to scope of training and service offered

- Increase in the ability to offer comprehensive care to the community, especially including emergency care

- Providing support to other disciplines and specialties, e.g. impending cardiac disease

- Contribution of skills and facilities required to deliver care to special populations

- Contribution to the multidisciplinary team approach in delivering care

- A resource for training in the variety of disciplines outside of dentistry

- Utilization of ancillary services thus helping to amortize costs

There are also financial benefits to the institution:

- The dental department is a revenue center which derives patient care income, Federal GME reimbursement, and a potential source of grant revenue from both government and private sources

As stated before, one of the keys to success depends on the chairperson's ability to forge a strong relationship with the senior administration and where possible, the members of the governing board.

Participation by the chairperson in activities which are important to top Administration is a significant sign of support which may reap substantial dividends in the long term. The Chairperson of the Dental Department also plays an advisory role within the institution and, in fact, functions as the in-house expert on all issues pertaining to dental matters. Interaction with the top Administration will provide visibility for the department can build allies for the department and will often inform the Chair of decisions regarding resource allocations. Similarly active participation with the medical staff can build important support for the department.

RELATIONSHIP TO MEDICAL STAFF

There are many facets to the relationship between the dental department and the medical staff.

a) The Department of Dental Medicine should enjoy equal status with all other clinical departments within the hospital. The Department therefore also shares equal responsibility as other departments. These responsibilities include staff responsibility for committee assignments as assigned by the Medical Executive Board, participation in clinical care activities and assistance in meeting regulatory activities. Dental services are especially in demand from Departments of Medicine (dialysis patients, oncology and cardiac care). As new scientific information becomes available, the need for interdepartmental collaboration which includes dentistry will be even more frequent.

b) Dental Residents rotate through medical departments in compliance with **CODA** standards.

Three major service areas link dental services with the medical staff. They are:

(1) EMERGENCY DEPARTMENT

The Emergency Department (ED) is one of the major portals of entry for the hospital. In many hospitals, it has become a very busy autonomous department with the Chairperson having a seat on the Medical Executive Board. Patients come to the Emergency Department most frequently as a result of trauma or infection. A number of these patients may require the services of the dental department, usually the Oral and Maxillofacial surgeon, but often enough the general dentistry resident may be first called to the ED. Performing dental services in the ED requires familiarity with policy and procedures of that department as well as the Protocols of the Department of Dental Medicine.

The conditions and requirements of service by dental staff in the ED are determined by agreement between the Chairpersons of Dentistry and the ED through the formulation of protocols and procedures which may be written, but are sometimes the result of oral agreements. Dental staff assigned to the ED, however, functions under the direction of the Chair of the ED during the period of assignment.

(2) ADMITTING

The Department of Dentistry treats inpatients, ambulatory surgery and same day surgery patients. Patients requiring general anesthesia, surgical patients, mentally and physically challenged patients, patients requiring the hospital environment because of medical complications comprise the patient load requiring the Admitting Department services.

Admission of dental patients involves coordination with the medical staff in conducting admitting physical examinations except in those cases where specific members of the dental staff have been granted admitting privileges.

(3) CONSULTATION

The consultation service was the original interface between dentistry and the hospitals. It remains a point of contact between the medical and dental staffs. Consultation services are a major source of patient referral among departments.

FACULTY, STAFF AND RESIDENCY RECRUITING

The chairperson is responsible for recruitment and hiring of all professional staff in accordance with the Medical Staff bylaws. The detailed policies for hiring are prescribed by the institution's Medical Staff Bylaws, the procedures as outlined by the Credentials Committee and the institution's Human Resources requirements. In addition, recruitment of staff should be determined by the needs of the department for service, teaching and administration.

The CODA document entitled "Accreditation Standards for Advanced Education Programs in General Practice Residency" provides general guidance with respect to faculty recruitment. Standard 3 describes the Program Director's responsibilities as including:

FACULTY AND STAFF (CODA STANDARD 3)

- Program administration
- Development and implementation of the curriculum plan
- Ongoing evaluation of program content, faculty teaching and resident performance
- Evaluation of resident training and supervision in affiliated institutions and off-services rotations
- Maintenance of records related to the educational program
- Resident selection

It is expected that program directors will devote sufficient time to accomplish the assigned duties and responsibilities. In programs where the program director assigns some duties to other individuals, it is expected that the program will develop a formal plan for such assignments that includes:

- What duties are assigned

- To whom they are assigned

- What systems of communication are in place between the program director and individuals who have been assigned responsibilities

In those programs where applicants are assigned centrally, responsibility for selection of residents may be delegated to a designee.

In hospitals where there is a clear distinction between the positions of chairperson and program director, the chairperson typically delegates the above listed responsibilities to the program director while retaining overall responsibility consistent with the chairperson's role. (See Appendix 1 & 2.)

Faculty members should be recruited in compliance with the minimum standards as outlined by CODA. They should, however, also demonstrate both interest and skill in teaching. Graduates of hospital programs (General Practice or Specialty) are preferred because of their familiarity with the somewhat arcane world of hospital practice. CODA standards require that "the program must be staffed by faculty who are qualified by education and/or clinical experience in the curriculum areas for which they are responsible and have collective competence in all areas of dentistry included in the program".

The program leadership is expected to develop criteria for hiring faculty. The standards require appropriate training (specialty qualification) or "current knowledge and appropriate levels of experience" for faculty. Departments are expected to develop written criteria which are used to certify a non-specialist, non-specialty qualified faculty member as qualified to teach. Teaching members of the attending staff are required to meet the criteria of the Credentials Committee of the institution, and obtain the approval of the Medical Executive Committee.

RESIDENCY RECRUITMENT

Residency recruiting has evolved from a random process prior to the nineteen eighties to a more formulaic one today. Many hospitals currently utilize the PASS and MATCH systems, both of which are voluntary. Most teaching hospitals employ specific pre-programmed steps in residency recruitment and appointment. During the eighties, the Match was adopted by most hospitals as part of the residency recruiting process. The "Match" was supposed to level the playing field for both applicant and institution. It was also supposed to be equitable for all participants and eliminate any existing exploitative elements.

Hospitals generally have specific processes for application to their programs. There may be, however, individual variations based on State requirements, institutional mission and attitude towards foreign graduates for example.

The goal of the residency recruitment process is the creation of a productive match between the institution and the applicant. This goal is best achieved when approached as a full disclosure process by both parties.

The department has a responsibility to disclose to applicants all information pertinent to the environment and culture of the department in addition to the program requirements and desired qualifications. In short, an institution's profile should be made available to applicants.

The interview process provides the opportunity for the department to discover the applicant's interests, potential and compatibility with the department policies and procedures. The interview should be a serious, probing event based on the understanding that interviews are a two-way street in which the applicant is making his/her own assessment of the leadership as well as the program, facilities, staff and other special characteristics.

The department has to be clear as to its own profile and must be able to present it in a comprehensible manner to applicants. The underlying principles in the recruitment process should be fairness and equity to the applicants.

It is recommended that each department maintains a written statement on residency selection which includes the application process, interview criteria and the interview process. It is also recommended that program directors appoint an advisory committee to assist in residency selection. The committee should play a role in screening applicants, reviewing applications, participate in the interview process and assist in ranking applicants. The use of an advisory committee demands development of agreed upon written selection criteria and calibration of interviewers.

Criteria specific to academic preparedness, clinical skill development and previous experience, should be objective. Other important attributes such as maturity, aptitude, communication skills, motivation and integrity are important to the selection process, but more difficult to measure, hence the need for careful calibration of interviewers.

Application Process

Whether or not the institution participates in the PASS system, hospitals require presentation of the applicant's transcript, academic records, National Board scores, Dean's letter of recommendation, two current recommendations of faculty or working associates and CV.

Interview Process

In addition to the above-mentioned recommendations, a specific interview period with limited dates is recommended. The dates selected should be convenient to the complete interviewing team. Candidates should be invited to visit the facility and meet with current Resident Staff prior to the scheduled interview.

It is my recommendation that interviews be conducted on a one-on-one basis, with interviewers comparing results and making selections based on established criteria. In a less than perfect world, this method is less intimidating and more efficient. Over the years, many applicants have described panel interviews involving multiple interviewers as disconcerting and confusing.

Resident Orientation

Resident orientation represents the first meaningful contact the resident has with the hospital. It is important, therefore, that the correct impression be created. Orientation must be carefully planned and executed. It sets the conditions of the hospital/residency relationship in a context that can be mutually beneficial to both parties. This period represents the transition from student to professional.

Careful planning and implementation will prove beneficial to both the applicant and the institution. Training programs and hospital services will be improved as a result of an effective orientation program.

The goals of the Orientation Program are:

- Reinforcement of the institutional and department mission
- Familiarizing the Resident with policies, procedures and protocols
- Introducing the new resident to personnel and their responsibilities
- Introduction to all Rules and Regulations
- Introduction to the institutional and department culture

- Topics covered would include infection control, child abuse reporting, Emergency codes, security, patient rights, performance improvement, OSHA standards, sexual harassment and due process. The list touches on key topics but is by no means complete.

Orientation programs are usually a combination of institution-specific and program-specific activities. Most residency programs conduct their own program-specific orientation.

There are key elements which lead to successful orientation. They are:

1. Good organization and preparation of all paperwork

2. Effective communication. Thought must be given to all aspects of communication. It must be appreciated that the sheer volume of information provided during orientation presents a challenge to the memory. Communication techniques should be employed, that will have both an immediate impact and lasting effect. Whenever feasible, hard copy should be provided to be used as a ready reference

3. Involve faculty. Faculty should be required to elucidate their goals, expectations and performance requirements. Written statements should supplement oral presentations. Such statements can be used to measure resident progress during the course of the residency (request biodata, immigration status, licensure contract and appointment agreement, delineation of privileges, CV).

4. Assure that all topics are covered including infection control practices, safety and security, radiology protection, HIPAA information, HIV confidentiality, others which may not be covered in institution-wide orientation.

5. Detailed review of the department Policy and Procedure manuals.

In general, adequate time should be allocated for each session to permit complete coverage of each topic including questions and answers.

CURRICULUM DEVELOPMENT

Standard 2-2 of the current CODA standards requires the program to have a curriculum plan. "The program is expected to organize the didactic and clinical educational experience into a formal curriculum plan."

Curriculum development is driven by the requirement of the Standards. Its goals are:

1. To permit the Resident to achieve competency in several prescribed areas.

2. To provide training in those areas at a level of skill and complexity beyond that achieved in pre-doctoral training.

3. To foster professional development of the resident.

The curriculum should emphasize professionalism, ethics, skill development, and appreciation of continuous learning, commitment to excellence, quality improvement, accountability and long term thinking. The curriculum should include all the learning experiences for which the institution assumes responsibility.

The Curriculum Plan should include:

*   Descriptions of training materials and modalities

*   Training content

*   Core training requirements

*   Plan for each year

*   Participation by trainees in the development of the curriculum. (It is important to know what not to teach). This is best identified by the trainees themselves. Effectiveness of the curriculum is measured by a system of outcomes assessment.

FINANCIAL MANAGEMENT

"Ever since general dentistry established its foothold in hospitals in the nineteen sixties, it has been under constant pressure to justify its tenancy——Dentistry's opportunity to grow and prosper is tied as closely to our ability to demonstrate our financial acumen and skill as it is tied to the ability to demonstrate the importance of our services to the institution and community".

These are the words of the author excerpted from a speech dating back to 1994. They are still all too often true today.

This is the point at which the "rubber hits the road". Financial management of hospitals has evolved from the primitive function of bookkeeping/accounting to a role in which it exerts a major influence in the management of hospital assets and the allocation of scarce resources.

Prior to the Medicaid legislation, the chief financial officer tended to be an accountant. Most accounting and budgeting virtually did not exist as hospital functions. Paralleling the progression to the corporate stage of hospital development, however, is the evolution of the role of the Chief Financial Officer into the second most important individual in the hierarchy. That individual is more concerned with managing information and planning creative solutions to problems than merely maintaining accounts.

It is my opinion that clinicians have not kept pace with the current trends in financial management. The result is that potential opportunities are not maximized and sources of friction develop with the administration of the hospital.

Budgeting

The budgeting process encompasses two dimensions: the human aspect and the business aspect. On the human side, the budget process

- Should be viewed as a tool by which the department can be improved.

- Requires management to both educate the Administration and to sell the department's program.

- Elicits natural human tendencies of resistance.

- Is an uphill process which is better developed as a bottom up rather than a top down tool.

The business objectives of a budget are:

- To provide a written expression of the plans in quantitative terms.

- To provide a basis for the evaluation of performance.

- To provide a useful tool for the control of costs.

- To create cost awareness throughout the department.

Budget development is a process and not just an event. The actual budget request must be written, should be well thought out, and should reflect the broad based thinking of the department in pursuing its goals. Ideally it is a bottom up rather than a top down process.

It is my experience that best results can be achieved by approaching the budget request in a manner similar to the style in which one approaches grant preparation; i.e., identifying a need, describing the method to be used for meeting the need, and then, establishing justifiable costs incurred as a result. Strong justification must be a part of the process.

Most hospitals use a "top-down" method of budgeting, by using the previous year's figures as a starting point and then adding some additional factor. This method of budgeting tends to constrain growth and innovation. "Bottom up budgeting", on the other hand, requires a demonstrable relationship between costs and benefits but does provide an opportunity for expansion. Regardless of the method, budget development results in a negotiating process among the key stakeholders.

In the days of "cost plus" reimbursement prior to the mid-eighties, there were five main cost influencing variables—case mix, number of cases, resources per case, input unit price and input efficiency. At that time clinicians exerted major control over only one of those variables, i.e. resources per case (mode of treatment).

In contrast, the subsequent Managed Care environment (since the nineties), requires clinicians to exert much greater influence and in some cases control over many more of those variables. Active financial management is now part of the Chairperson's responsibility and involves decisions that go well beyond control of treatment mode. It includes greater responsibility for other variables. Independent revenue enhancement and fundraising are now an expectation of department leadership. Grants have been the traditional source of non patient income. Other sources must be considered, such as philanthropic, research and commercial support.

Budgeting is a process which involves three distinct but equally important tasks. First, the budget should be prepared; second, the budget should be written, and finally, the budget should be monitored.

GRADUATE MEDICAL EDUCATION

Any discussion of financial management must include an understanding of the funding of Graduate Medical Education (GME). The federal government plays an important role in the funding of hospital sponsored Residency training through the Medicare program. Specific formulas are applied to direct and indirect costs.

An understanding of direct and indirect costs incurred by the department, how they are assigned or allocated and their impact on the overall institutional finances is required. Funds derived from Medicare under the Graduate Medical Education reimbursement formula impacts the teaching hospital's overall budget. The amounts involved are substantial and are of high value to the hospital.

GME funds are paid directly to the hospital and not to the department. Some institutions credit the department with a portion of the funds. Since this reimbursement is based on residency positions, the value of dental residency programs is enhanced to the extent that they train Residents. In 1997 the federal government froze the number of approved residency programs nationally. Dental residencies were exempted from the cap.

The reimbursement formula, rules and regulations, change periodically. It is therefore useful for department chairmen to have some understanding of the rules related to GME funding.

Prior to passage of the Medicare and Medicaid legislation (Titles 18 and 19), individual hospitals and their supporting communities bore the costs of residency programs by direct funding of medical education. During the 1960s, a projected shortage of physicians to meet an increasing demand for health services led to the federal government assuming substantial financial responsibility for paying for medical education.

As a result, reimbursement for resident costs is provided by the federal government under terms defined by Congress. This arrangement has been controversial and subject to change. Every chairperson should therefore be familiar with its terms on a current basis. A brief look at the methodology of GME reimbursement reveals that it is allocated in two parts: first, Direct Reimbursement, which covers the direct costs associated with residency such as resident salaries, stipends and benefits, faculty salaries, administrative costs and others directly incurred by the residency program. The second part is a more complex, periodically changing formula which covers (other costs) by relating to a resident to bed ratio. In summary, Indirect Medical Education reimbursement is based upon three components:

- Per resident amount

- Full Time Equivalent Resident counts eligible for payment

- Medicare Utilization based upon inpatient days

Prior to 1983 GME was cost reimbursed and based on whatever was spent by the hospital. Subsequent to that date GME has been subject to several legislative and regulatory changes.

GME reimbursement is limited to hospitals and is not available to dental schools except under special circumstances.

These changes are designed to reduce costs and cap the numbers of Residents. At this time of writing, dental residents have been exempt from restrictions of the cap.

Acts which modified/and or changed GME include:

- BBA—Balance Budget Act 1997

- BBRA—Balanced Budget Refinement Act HR3426 (1999)

- BIPA—Benefits and Improvement Act HR5661 (2000)

Given the volatility of GME regulations it behooves the leadership of the dental department to remain informed about the changes occurring in GME regulations.

PERFORMANCE IMPROVEMENT/QUALITY ASSURANCE

The Institute of Medicine (IOM) in 1990 defined Quality as the degree to which health services increase desired health outcomes and are consistent with current professional knowledge. The concept of Quality Improvement (QI) gained considerable impetus with publication of the Institute of Medicine (IOM) report in 1999. Its roots, however, go back much further to the writing of Donabedian and others who, in the late 1970s, began to elaborate on the topic of evaluation in health care. He enunciated the now classic "structure", "process", "outcome" model for assessment of quality of care. He envisaged this model as being effective in linking quality, access and cost in health care.

During the 1980s and 1990s, under the influence of Deming and Juran, the concept of continuous Quality Improvement made its way into the commercial sector of the country. As part of the 'corporatization' of hospitals, performance improvement was adopted by hospitals as an important function requiring a symbiotic relationship between the medical/dental staff and Administration. The importance of QI is reinforced by the fact that all payors—government, insurance, and private individuals are now demanding greater accountability for their expenditures.

Consumers are also demanding assured quality care and hospitals are now subject to report cards. [A point of clarification in terminology—Quality Improvement (QI) is systems oriented, Quality Assurance (QA) is oriented to individuals.]

The importance of Quality Improvement requires that the dental unit (department or service) be actively involved in the hospital-wide system in addition to departmental activities. It is important that Residents be taught the concepts and be equipped with the tools to manage quality. The General Practice Residency Standards require Residents participation in QA.

Cunningham and Motaro have outlined a process which is applicable to dental departments. Their process describes a hierarchy which includes "Quality Control," "Quality Assurance", "Continuous quality improvement," "Outcomes management," "clinical process improvement."

Quality control describes the routine repeat monitoring of the functioning of equipment, supplies and procedures related to their use. Examples of activities suitable for quality control include:

- Biological testing of autoclaves
- Testing of lead aprons and film badges
- Monitoring of anesthesia equipment
- Monitoring of medication expiration dates
- Preventive maintenance of clinical equipment
- Monitoring of x-ray machine performance
- Radiation and biohazard exposure testing

Quality Assurance is the next level in the hierarchy in which direct care provided by clinicians is evaluated. Under this rubric the structures and processes of health care are measured. The department selects the aspects of care which are to be measured and also selects the QA indicators to be measured. The framework requires the department to set (a) Standards of Care covering patient experience,

(b) Standards of Practice covering dentist performance and (c) Threshold Standards to be met, usually expressed as percentage compliance.

Continuous Quality Improvement is a more objective data-based assessment of a selected process from a quality assurance. It is a systematic review of a clearly identified process with the view of continuously improving the process utilizing a formal review process. Unlike QA there are no thresholds to be met.

QUALITY ASSURANCE/OUTCOMES ASSESSMENTS

Outcome Assessments

Outcomes Assessments (OA) evaluation is an important mandate of CODA. OA requires documentation as a means of measuring what is learned instead of what is taught. Outcomes are expressed in terms of predetermined proficiency or competencies.

Assessment includes departmental outcomes as well as individual and program outcomes. It requires a systematic and consistent approach based on steps made explicit to all involved parties: residents, faculty and rotation chiefs. Outcomes assessment should be an important element of the continuous quality improvement process. OA is based on four concepts which are:

1. Plan
2. Do
3. Check
4. Act

These same principles may be expressed in different terminology according to differing authorship.

OUTREACH

Outreach programs represent an important activity of many hospitals. In some instances the dental department may develop independent outreach activities associated exclusively with the department. When properly designed they satisfy the CODA requirement for training in community health. They also extend the service capabilities of the department and in those instances in which they are well planned can prove to be effective marketing tools. They are also a positive public relations tool for the hospital. Among the many opportunities for outreach programs are the following:

- Health fairs—the most common activity
- Cancer screening (joint programs especially continuing education))
- Developmentally disabled programs
- Dental Societies (joint programs especially continuing education)
- Nursing homes programs
- School-based projects
- Miscellaneous service and education opportunities e.g. mobile service vans

SAMPLE DENTAL MANUAL

Section 1

Introduction

- Mission
- Program Description

Section 2

Goals and Objectives

Section 3

Organization of Program

- Table of Organization
- Rotation
- On call
- Position Description
- Chief Resident Responsibility

Section 4

General Information & Regulations

Library Resources

- Attendance at lectures, conferences, seminars
- Quality assurance
- Resident log

Section 5

Patient Management

- Radiological Examination
- Chart Completion
- Diagnosis and Treatment Planning
- Responsibility for Patients
- Scheduling of Patients Load
- Management of Emergencies
- Management of Broken Appointments
- Recall System
- Use of Conscious Sedation
- Completion of Treatment

Section 6

Dental Emergency Room coverage

Inpatient Consultations

Section 7

Care of Dental Inpatients and Ambulatory Surgery Patients

- Establish need for hospitalization
- Admission procedures
- Patient workup

- Patient rounds
- Preoperative procedures
- OR protocol
- Operating room procedures
- Post-operative orders
- Discharge Procedures

Section 8

Overview of Curriculum/outcomes

- Assignment to other services/rotations
- Anesthesiology rotation
- Ambulatory/Preadmission rotation
- Emergency department rotation
- Endodontics
- Implant surgery
- Operative dentistry
- Oral Surgery
- Orthodontic Protocol
- Pathology
- Pediatric Dentistry
- Periodontal protocol
- Prevention & health promotion
- Prosthetics

Section 9

Quality Assurance Program

Section 10

Evaluation

Policy re: summary of Competencies

Section 11

Grievance procedure process

Policy re: grievances procedure process

Due process

Section 12

General

- Infection control laboratory procedures
- Equipment care and maintenance
- Community Service
- Outreach activities, dress and deportment
- Newsletter.

REGULATIONS

There is a plethora of external agencies which regulate the operations of hospitals. Regulations may originate from federal, state and local governments. Some regulations have a direct bearing on the operation of the dental department. Prominent among these agencies are the American Dental Association (ADA), the Joint Commission *(JCAHO), the Occupational Safety and Health Administration Act (OSHA), Health Resources and Services Administration. (HRSA).

The American Dental Association (ADA) is the professional body which sets standards, provides dental technical information, political and regulatory information for the profession. CODA sets the standards and accredits the GPR, AEGD and other training programs which are sponsored by institutions.

JCAHO is a nonprofit organization established in 1951, having an important role in establishing the standards of health care delivery in the USA. Its stated mission is to improve the quality of care provided to the public. The Commission performs this function through the mechanism of periodic announced and sometimes unannounced site surveys which result in approvals or disapprovals. JCAHO decisions play an important role in hospital reimbursement.

OSHA was established in 1970. Its mission is to prevent work-related injuries, illness and death by issuing and enforcing standards for workplace safety and health. Because the dental profession utilizes complex equipment and many potentially hazardous materials, OSHA and its subsidiaries play a significant role in a dental department. Implementation of universal precautions falls under OSHA's purview.

HIPAA is federal legislation covering the area of individual health insurance plans. The legislation includes multiple titles. The dental department is most affected by title 11 which covers the Privacy Rule. This rule establishes regulations for the use and disclosure of Protected Health Information. (PHI). PHI is any information about health status, provision of health care or payment for health care that can be linked to an individual. This regulation covers any part of an individual patient's medical record or payment history.

HRSA is the division of the Department of Health and Human Services that seeks to promote access to care for vulnerable populations such as the uninsured, the physically isolated, the medically uninsured, the HIV population, other special needs populations and maternal and child health populations. Together with the National Institutes of Health (NIH), HRSA is a primary funding agency for training and research grants. HRSA administers grants for general practice residencies, pediatric dental residencies, among several others.

AIDS/HIV Programs And Public Health Training programs. This agency has been very important to hospital dentistry over the past thirty years. In addition to the above-mentioned agencies, state governments do exercise regulatory control through the mechanisms of licensures, certification of all dental providers, in some states the issuance of temporary permits. Local governments regulate infrastructure issues e.g. the issuing of occupancy certificates and inspecting radiology equipment.

APPENDIXES

APPENDIX 1

Job Title: Chairperson
Department: Dentistry Department

Principal Duties and Responsibilities:

He/She is a fulltime Educational and Administrative Officer of the Department of Dentistry.

a. He/She is responsible for the organization and operation of the department and for the work of the staff of the department. The Director may examine any patient and recommend a course of treatment.

b. The Chairperson is a member of the Executive Committee of the Medical Board giving guidance on the overall medical policies of the hospital and making specific recommendations regarding his/her own department to assure quality patient care.

c. The Chairperson maintains continuing review of the professional performance of all dentists on the staff.

d. The Chairperson has overall responsibility for the training and Education program in the department.

e. He/she participates in every phase of administration of the department, including matters of patient care, personnel, supplies, special regulations and techniques.

f. Serves on appropriate committees of the Medical Board as an elected or appointed member.

g. Responsible for coordinating activities involving dental care with other departments in the hospital.

h. He/she participates directly in the education program

i. Prepares and monitors budget

j. Responsible for strategic planning

k. Responsible for fundraising

APPENDIX 2

Program director

3-1 The program director must have authority and responsibility for all aspects of the program.

Intent: The program director's responsibilities include:

    a.   programs administration

    b.   development and implementation of the curriculum plan

    c.   ongoing evaluation of program content, faculty teaching and student/ resident performances

    d.   evaluation of student/resident training and supervision in affiliated institution and services rotation

    e.   maintenance of records related to the educational program

    f.   student/resident selection

It is expected that the program directors will devote sufficient time to accomplish the assigned duties and responsibilities. In programs where the program director assigns some duties to other individuals, it is expected that the program will develop a formal plan for assignments that include:

1. what duties are assigned

2. to whom they are assigned

3. what systems of communication are in place between the program director and individuals who have assigned responsibilities

APPENDIX 3

History and Authority of the Commission:

The Commission of Dental Accreditation, the successor of the Council on Dental Education which had conducted the accreditation program since 1937, began operating in 1975. The Commission serves as the only nationally recognized accrediting body for dentistry and the related dental fields. The Commission receives its accreditation authority from the acceptance of dental community and by being recognized by the U.S. Department of education (USDOE) and by the Commission on Recognition of Postsecondary Accreditation (CORPA).

Recognition by a voluntary, non-governmental agency, such as CORPA and its predecessor, the Council on Postsecondary Accreditation (COPA), represents respect for basicprinciples of institution authority and adherence in other good accreditation practices. The commission has participated in non-governmental recognition since 1964.

Eligibility for federal funding is linked to recognition by the USDOE, a governmental agency. Statutory restrictions mandate that educational institution or programs must be accredited by USDOE-recognized accrediting agency (often called a "gatekeeper") in order to be eligible for federal funding. The Commission has participated in governmental recognition since 1954.

Both CORPA and USDOE have established recognition requirements that an accrediting agency must meet in order to be recognized. Both agencies typically conduct reviews for recognition at five-year intervals.

Dental Accreditation: Historical Perspective

The American Dental Association (ADA) authorized the Council of Dental Education to accredit dental schools in 1938; however the Requirements of Approval of a Dental School did not go into effect until the 1941–1942 school year. The Council's initial accrediting activities were confined to dental schools. As the dental profession developed and grew, however, the scope of accrediting activities also grew. Current activities include accreditation of dental programs for dental assistants, dental hygienists and dental laboratory technicians, as well as accreditation for advanced programs for general dentistry, the eight recognized dental specialties and general practice residences, in addition to predictor al education programs.

In 1973, House of Delegates of the American Dental Association approved the establishment of a commission of accreditation of Dental and Dental Auxiliary Education Programs. In 1979 this body's name was officially changed to the Commission of Dental Accreditation. The twenty (20) member Commission includes the twelve (12) Council of Dental Education members, four of whom represent the American Dental Association, four (4) the American Association of Dental Examiners and four for the American Association of Dental Schools. The additional eight (8) Commission representatives include two (2) dental specialists selected by specialty organizations having certifying boards recognized by the association, one (1) representative selected by the American Dental Assistants Association, one (1) representative from the American Hygienists Association, one (1) certified dental laboratory technician selected by the National Association of Dental Laboratories, one (1) student representative selected jointly by the American Student Dental Association and the Council of Students of American Association of Dental Schools and two (2) public representatives elected by the Council of Dental Education.

In the event a commission member sponsoring organization fails to select a Commissioner, the Council on Dental Education selects an appropriate representative to serve as a Commissioner, as specified in Rules.

Source:

Evaluation Policies and Procedures, American Dental Association. Commission on Dental Accreditation, Chicago 1996.

APPENDIX 4

SAMPLE ATTENDING EVALUATION OF RESIDENT FORM

Resident's Name _____ Evaluator's Name _____

Evaluation period _____

Directions: For each item please write the number which best corresponds to your evaluation of the individual. Please write any comments you may have under the advice and comment section or on the back of this page if necessary.

Rating Scale   5= Truly Exceptional   4= Advanced   3= Proficient
              2= Needs Remediation   1= Unsatisfactory   0= Not Observed

I. General Professional Conduct   COMMENTS

1.   Demonstrated effective interpersonal relations

2.   Displayed sensitivity to peers, staff and patients

3.   Elicited suitable patient reactions

4.   Exhibited proper decorum (etiquette)

5.   Demonstrated responsibility

6.   Accepted constructive criticism

7.   Sought help when needed

8.   Actively sought patient care opportunities

II. Patient Management

1.   Gathered appropriate H and P information

2.   Prioritized patient needs

3.   Developed appropriate treatment plans (drugs, treatment, consult)

4.   Demonstrated appropriate dental knowledge

5.   Demonstrated good clinical judgment

6.   Promoted preventative care

7. Identified biopsychosocial issues

8. Communicated with clarity (oral and written)

9. Participated in discussion

10. Inferred adequate differential diagnoses

11. Adapted treatment plan according to patient's social/psychological background

III. **Knowledge and Skills**

1. Demonstrated an adequate range and depth of knowledge

2. Demonstrated knowledge of basic science (clinical correlations)

3. Communicated with clarity (oral and written)

4. Participated in discussion

IV. **Resident Case Presentation**

1. Identified educational needs at the beginning of the interaction

2. Presented accurate, complete information

3. Presented cases in a logical manner

4. Drew accurate conclusions

SAMPLE ATTENDING EVALUATION OF RESIDENT IN OUTPATIENT SETTING

Resident's Name(s) _____ Evaluator's Name _____

Clinic _____ Evaluation Period _____

Directions: For each item in Section 1—1V, please write the number that best corresponds to your evaluation of the individual. For each item in section V, circle or write response. Please write any comments you have under the advice and comment section or on the back of the page if necessary.

Rating Scale: 5 = Always   4 = Often   3 = Occasionally

                 2 = Rarely   1 = Never   0 = No information

1. General Professional Conduct   **COMMENTS**

1. Demonstrated effective interpersonal relations

2. Exhibited proper decorum (etiquette)

3. Exhibited enthusiasm

4. Accepted constructive criticism and advice

5. Dictated succinct, complete description of visit

6. Formulated appropriate medical diagnosis and treatment plan

7. Maintained flowsheet

8. Documented follow-up

V. **Communication and Observation**

How often did the resident consult you daily?   0 1 2 3 4 5 5+

How often did you initiate contact with the resident

on a daily basis?   0 1 2 3 4 5 5+

Did you observe the resident by video?   Yes___ No ___

How often did you observe the resident with the patient? 0 1 2 3 4 5 5+

The resident's OVERALL performance was

___ Truly Exceptional   __ Advanced   ___ Proficient
___ Needs Remediation __ Unsatisfactory ___ Incomplete

Advice and comments:

PROGRAM EVALUATION TEMPLATE
Resident Evaluation

All information should be stored in evaluation folders/portfolios for each individual.

Database of aggregate data should be maintained for program evaluation.

1. Before entry into the program, resident applicants

   a. Review letters of recommendation, dean's letter, board scores, comments made by interviewers; assure licensure is attainable and granted.

   b. When a resident applicant is given a patient care scenario, residency faculty assess each applicant's ability to diagnose and manage based on information given.

   c. Residents entering the program with advanced standing (prior credit) need additional official documentation and must apply in an ethical manner.

   d. Assess interpersonal skills.

   e. Identify applicants' demographics which would predict those individuals interested in a specific specialty, and select applicants accordingly.

2. Academic Year

   a. First month

      Self-Assessment knowledge base, attitude and skills.

   b. Each month/rotation

      1. Evaluation by attending faculty

   b. Every three months

   c. 1. Chart audits review

      2. Procedure/diagnosis documentation reviewed

      3. Patient satisfaction questionnaires reviewed

      4. Rotation evaluation by faculty, staff and fellow residents reviewed

      5. Individual resident goals and progress towards goals reviewed

6, Practices styles reviewed

7. Conference attendance and conference presentation reviewed

SAMPLE LECTURE EVALUATION FORM

Speaker's Name _____ Date _____

Topic _____

Directions: for each item, please write the number which best corresponds to your evaluation. Please write any comments you may have under the comment section or on the back of this page if necessary.

Rating   Scale: 5 = Strongly Agree   4 = Agree   3 = Neutral   2 = Disagree
1 = Strongly Disagree   0 = Not Applicable

COMMENTS:

1.   The lecture provided me with new information

2.   The presentation contained information appropriate to my level of training

3.   The presenter seemed organized and prepared

4.   The presenter answered questions clearly and concisely

5.   The presenter engaged the residents by asking questions

6.   The presenter was enthusiastic

7.   The presenter used examples and illustrations to explain and clarify

8.   The presenter used AV materials and handouts efficiently

9.   The lecture objectives were met

10. Overall the lecturer taught me effectively

Additional Comments

Your Name (optional) _____

REFERENCES

1. Hazlewood, Arthur I. "Hospital governance, Administration and Organization", Hospital Dentistry Practise and Education, rd Raymond F. Zambito. Harold A. Black and Lorraine B. Tesch (St. Louis: Mosby 1996) 7–26

2. Wheatley, Margaret J. Leadership and the New Science. Discovering Order in a Chaotic World 3rd. ed. Bernett-Koehler Publishers, Inc. 2006

3. United States Army Infantry School, United States Artillery Handbook ST 7-163FY73, United States Army Fort Benning. Ga. 1973

4. Hazlewood Arthur I. Speech, financial Assessment of Hospital Dental Practices, Federation Special Care Dentistry, Washington, D.C. 1994

5. Glover, J.D, Chief Executive's Handbook. Homewood, IL: Dow Jones Irwin Inc 19765; 304

6. Donabedian, A., 1988 The Quality of Care. How can it be assessed? Journal of the American Medical Association; 260: 743-1748.

7. Denning, W. Edwards Management at Work N.Y. 1990

8. Juran, Joseph, Quality Control Handbook 1988.

Suggested Readings

Demb A. Neubauer FF: The corporate board, NY 1992, Oxford University Press.

Griffith JR: The well managed community hospital, ed 2, Ann Arbor, Mich, 1992, Health Administration Press.

Humble M: Duties, responsibilities and liability of directors of non profit health care institutions, La Jolla, California, 1994, Governance Institute.

Landgarten S: The board's responsibility for quality in a managed care marketplace, La Jolla, Calif, 1995, Governance Institute

McGybony JR: Principles of hospital administration, ed 2, NY, 1969, GP Putnam's Sons

Pointer DD, Ewell CM: Really governing: how health system and hospital boards can make more of a difference, NY, 1994 Delmar Press.

Pruyser: PW: The minister as diagnostician, Philadelphia, 1976, Westminster Press.

Cryer MH: history of the organization of oral surgical staff of the Philadelphia Hospital, Appendix G, Phila Gen Hosp Rep 5: 17–18, 1902

Weinberger BW: An introduction to the history of dentistry in America, St. Louis, 1948 Mosby

Zambito RF, Lemmey C: Establishing and managing a hospital dental department, Part 1 and 11, Quintessence Int 5:8–12, 1984; 5:1 7, 1986

MacEachern MD: Hospital organization and management, ed 3, Berwyn, Ill, 1957, Physicians Record.

Goldberg, AJ, Buttaro RA: Hospital department profiles, ed 3 Chicago, 1990, Applied Management Systems for Healthcare Information and Management Systems Society of the American Hospital Association.

RESOURCES

Bass, Bernard (1989) Stogdill's Handbook of Leadership: A survey of theory and Research. NY: Free Press

Bolman, L. and Deal, T. (1991) Reframing Organizations: San Francisco: Jossey-Bass.

Kouzes, James M. & Posner, Barry Z. (1987) The Leadership Challenge San Francisco: Jossey-Bass

U.S.A. Handbook (1973) Military Leadership

Wasserman, Burton S. (2007) CQI Corner-Credentialing Special Care Dentistry Newsletter Jan-Feb. 2007

Association for Hospital Medical Education. Guide to Graduate Medical Education 2nd ed. (1998) Washington, D.C.

Juran JM, Gryna FM: Juran's quality control handbook, ed 4, New York 1988 McGraw-Hill.

Walton N: Deming management at work, New York, 1990, Perigree.

GUIDE TO WEB SITES

Accreditation Council for Graduate Medical Education

www.acgme.org

American Dental association

www.ada.org

American Hospital Association

www.aha.org

American Medical Association

www.ama.org

American Dental Education Association

www.adea.org

Centers for Medicare and Medicaid Services

www.cmh.hhs.gov

Department of Health and Human Services

www.dhhs.gov

Journal of American Medical Association

www.Jama.ama-assn.org

Academy of General Dentistry

www.agd.org

Health Resources and Services Administration

www.hrsa.gov

International and American Association for Dental Research

www.iadr.com

National Institute of Dental and Craniofacial Research

   www.nidcr.nih.gov

National Institutes of Health

   www.nih.gov

National Dental Association

   www.ndaonline.org

National Maternal and Child Oral Health Resource Center

   www.mcoralhealth.org

United States Public Health Services

   www.his.gov

Institute of Medicine

   www.iom.edu

Joint Commission on Accreditation of Health Care Organizations

   www.jcaho.org

978-0-595-46883-6
0-595-46883-7